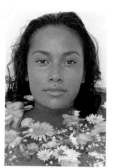

healing with
flowers

a concise guide

to using flowers

to balance the mind,

body and emotions

Jessica Houdret

HERMES
HOUSE

The edition published by Hermes House

© Anness Publishing Limited 2002 updated 2003..

Hermes House is an imprint of Anness Publishing Limited,
Hermes House, 88–89 Blackfriars Road, London SE1 8HA

Publisher: Joanna Lorenz
Production Controller: Joanna King

Publisher's Note:

The Reader should not regard the recommendations, ideas and techniques
expressed and described in this book as substitutes for the advice of a
qualified medical practitioner or other qualified professional.
Any use to which the recommendations, ideas and techniques
are put is at the reader's sole discretion and risk.

Printed in Hong Kong/China

3 5 7 9 10 8 6 4

contents

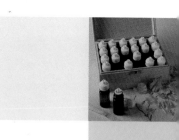

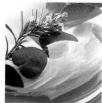

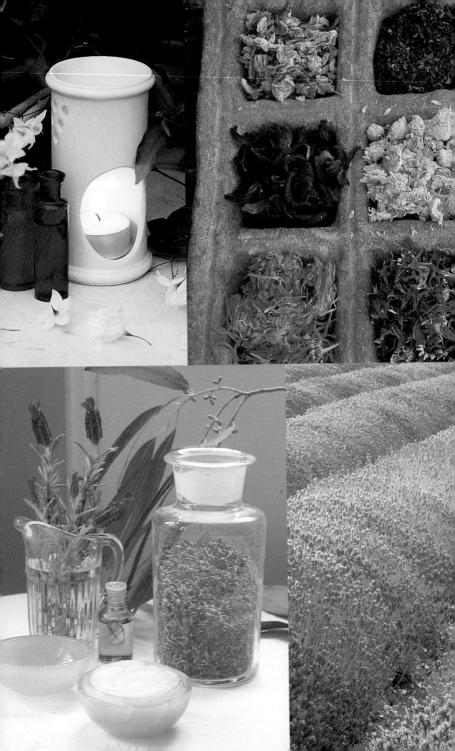

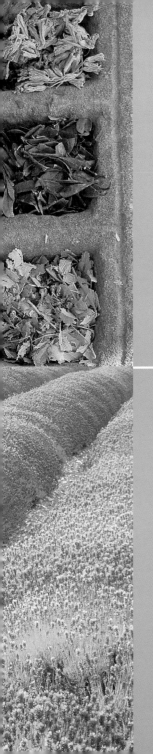

introduction

Healing with flowers and herbs is as ancient as mankind, and for most of human history was the only medical option available. Even today, it is estimated that three-quarters of our pharmaceutical drugs are plant-based.

There has been a huge recent revival of interest in flower healing, and medical research is proving that plant remedies are indeed highly effective.

The following pages describe how to harvest, dry, prepare and store healing flowers; they explain how to make flower teas, tinctures, infusions, compresses and inhalants; and a directory of 60 healing flowers introduces some of the most useful plants available.

History of healing with flowers

Until the advent of pharmaceutically based medicine at the beginning of the 19th century, healing systems in all cultures relied upon plants. Indeed, many of today's manufactured pills were originally made from plants.

EARLY HEALING SYSTEMS

Many ancient civilizations had well-developed medicinal plant healing systems. The earliest recorded natural healing methods were in China nearly 5,000 years ago, but because China remained closed to the West for many centuries, it is the texts recorded on tablets and papyri from the early civilizations of Sumeria and Egypt which are the antecedents of the later European healers. The great physicians of ancient Greece – Hippocrates, Galen, Theophrastus and Dioscorides – drew on these earlier cultures when writing their own works.

The name of Paracelsus (1493–1541), a 16th-century Swiss physician and alchemist, stands out in particular. He declared that he had not taken his knowledge from the Greek

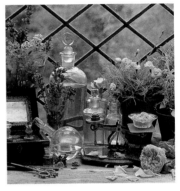

▲ FLOWERS HAVE BEEN USED FOR HEALING PURPOSES THROUGHOUT HISTORY.

"father of medicine" Hippocrates, the influential Roman physician Galen or anyone else, but "from the best teachers: experience and hard work". Paracelsus believed that disease originated from a departure with essential spirituality, and that by balancing the four elements, a substance called a "quintessence" was created, which healed the soul. The right essence, whether of a flower or mineral, would renew the connection with the spirit within, which was the true healer.

THE RENAISSANCE

From earliest times there has been a belief in the power of flower fragrance to protect from disease. This led to the 15th-century production of pomanders, the use of posies, strewing herbs and herbal fumigation. Diet was also considered integral to healing – herbs and flowers were added to food for their medicinal action as much as for their nutritional or flavouring capabilities.

THE MODERN ERA

In the early 19th century, the medical establishment moved away from remedies made with plants to laboratory-produced chemical drugs. This was a great step forward for civilization as general health improved and cures were found for many diseases, but a side-effect was that much of the responsibility for their own minor health problems was taken out of the hands of ordinary people and home remedies began to be forgotten.

During the last century Edward Bach (1886–1936), the founder of modern flower essence therapy, pioneered the treatment

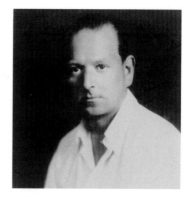

▲ EDWARD BACH, PIONEER OF MODERN FLOWER REMEDIES.

of the whole person by using safe and natural remedies. Of Welsh origin, Bach was born in Birmingham and trained as a bacteriologist. Later, in 1919, he joined the staff of the London Homeopathic Hospital.

Bach believed that for healing to succeed, the emotions, particularly fear, uncertainty and shock had to be addressed in depth. By 1928, he was experimenting with flowers, finding that impatiens, clematis and mimulus worked well to calm certain mental states.

Much ancient plant lore has recently been revived in the use of flowers in both internal and external forms of self-healing.

Using flowers to heal

 The ways in which you can use flowers to heal include inhaling uplifting flower scents, drinking soothing teas, unwinding with a relaxing flower oil massage, or allowing the subtle energy of a flower essence to work on your deepest emotions.

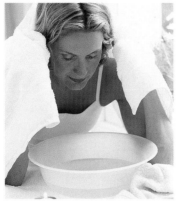

FLOWER OILS

Essential oils extracted from flowers have a powerful effect on mental and emotional states. Breathing in their vapours can be relaxing, restorative or uplifting. One way to inhale the scent is simply to put a few drops on a handkerchief and keep it on your pillow overnight. But for a more controlled and concentrated method, which is also longer lasting, an essential oil burner is ideal. Other ways of benefiting from oils include adding a few drops to a warm bath, or diluting and massaging into the skin.

FLOWER TEAS

Also known as tisanes, flower teas have been used for medicinal purposes for many centuries. Lavender, hyssop and thyme were taken to alleviate cold symptoms, while chamomile and lime flower were used against insomnia. Whatever the virtues, the scent of these tisanes alone is a tonic and they can be enjoyed simply for this reason.

FLOWER TONICS

Plants that affect the nervous system interact powerfully with the body. These are known as nervines, and invigorate and nourish the whole nervous system. Restorative nervine tonics include St John's wort, sage and mugwort. Relaxing tonics include skullcap, vervain and wood betony.

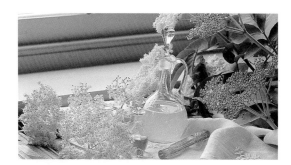

◀ YOU CAN STORE YOUR HOME-MADE FLOWER REMEDIES IN ORNATE BOTTLES.

FLOWER ESSENCES

Natural flower remedies do not address the organs of our bodies, like our heart, liver and lungs, and their ailments. Rather, the remedies work on basic mental and emotional states.

Recent research suggests that water has a "memory" and can hold the imprint of a flower's properties, passing these on to us. Bach himself made sun-potentized flower essences in pure water.

Just as beautiful music can inspire us and help us feel whole, so can flower essences, Bach said. Some people now use the term "vibrational medicine" to make the analogy between music and the flowers clearer.

▶ THE SEPARATE COMPARTMENTS OF THIS SPECIALLY DESIGNED ESSENCE BOX KEEP THEIR INDIVIDUAL HEALING PROPERTIES CLEAR.

So, if our particular challenge is the anger or jealousy aspect of oversensitivity, holly essence will encourage acceptance of the emotion and bring out our love and tolerance. If the struggle is with the discouragement aspect of uncertainty, gentian essence can revive our courage and faith.

There is no harm in taking flower essences along with herbal tonics or essential oils, herb teas, aromas or inhalants. Each of these are healing expressions of the positive power of herbs and plants.

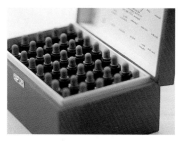

Flower cultivation

The process of cultivating, harvesting, drying and storing flowers can be a healing experience in itself. It is also the best way to learn the qualities of many remarkable healing plants, although buying flowers also gives good results.

GROWING

It is relatively easy to grow healing flowers, partly because many of these plants are wild in origin and do not suffer much from pests and diseases. Their aromatic smells often keep away harmful insects.

Cultivating your own healing flowers means you know exactly what has been put on them, and you can choose to go organic, using compost or mulches if you wish. Since many healing flowers are considered to be weeds — including red clover, horehound,

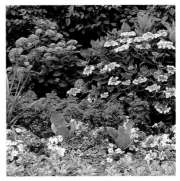

▲ MANY OF THE PLANTS FOUND IN GARDENS TODAY HAVE BEEN USED FOR THEIR HEALING PROPERTIES FOR 2,000 YEARS.

elder, selfheal and yarrow of those listed in the directory at the end of the book — they actually thrive on neglect and can colonize otherwise unused land.

HARVESTING

Reaping the flowers is a continuous rather than a one-off process. Most plants will be vigorous enough to allow repeated picking in small amounts, which encourages their further growth. It is best to gather flowers, stems and leaves when they are at their

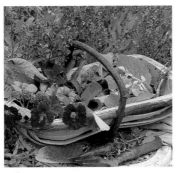

▲ GATHER FLOWERS IN THE MORNING, WHEN THE SUN HAS CAUSED THE DEW TO EVAPORATE AND ENCOURAGED THE FRAGRANCE TO DEVELOP.

peak, which for flowers means on a sunny morning and for leaves before flowering begins. Roots should be dug up in the autumn, cleaned and chopped into small pieces.

If gathering wild flowers, be sure you have identified the plant correctly. Use a wild flower book, and pick them away from busy roads. Many wild plants are protected by law and should be left alone.

DRYING

In order to dry flowers and herbs successfully, the moisture needs to be removed without losing the plant's volatile oils. Natural drying in an airing cupboard that is well ventilated is good. Loosely

▶ HANG BUNCHES OF FLOWERS UPSIDE DOWN TO DRY.

sealed brown paper bags can be used for drying small quantities. Using an oven even at a low setting is usually too hot for flowers and leaves, although it may be needed for roots.

STORING

Keep dried flowers and herbs in separate airtight containers in the dark, and label and date them. If hanging bundles, keep them in a dry, airy place out of the sunlight. If you prefer, store freshly gathered plants in the freezer. This method works well for lemon balm and parsley, which lose their flavour when dried. Tinctures are used to preserve selected herbs in alcohol.

BUYING

If buying flowers is your preference, choose ones that seem fresh, and which have retained their colour and aroma.

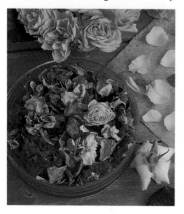

◀ DRIED ROSE PETALS MAKE A COLOURFUL AND FRAGRANT POTPOURRI WHICH CAN HELP TO PROMOTE A FEELING OF WELLBEING.

Flower preparation

Flowers should be gathered on a warm dry morning, before the sun has become too strong and drawn out the essential oils. They are best picked in bud or freshly opened, when their scent and flavour are at their most enticing.

GATHERING FLOWERS

Those who are allergic to pollen should not eat flowers. In any case, it is still best to cut out the central reproductive areas, where the stamens and pollen are to be found, if you can. Individual flowers vary greatly but some, such as lilies and hibiscus, are particularly heavy with pollen and it is obvious which parts should be removed. With smaller flowers such as primroses, cowslips, violas and marjoram this would be difficult in the extreme, so if anyone is susceptible to allergy it is best to avoid all flowers.

Separate the petals from the green parts surrounding them – it is easier in some plants, such as marigolds, than others, such as violets or hollyhocks. Plants that flower in umbels, such as fennel, are best used whole.

▼ MAKE SURE THAT YOU IDENTIFY WILD FLOWERS CORRECTLY BEFORE PICKING THEM.

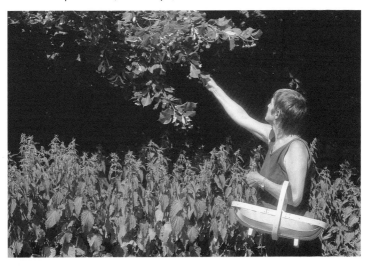

The body can benefit from the healing properties of flowers by using treatments both internally and externally.

INTERNAL USES

Flowers can be taken internally in infusions, inhalations, tinctures, teas, as capsules and powders, and in the many different types of preparations used to flavour and enhance cooking.

EXTERNAL USES

Flowers can be used externally in compresses, poultices, ointments, potpourris, skin creams, infused oils, massage and bath oils.

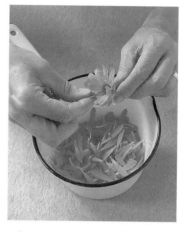

▲ CREAMS MADE FROM POT MARIGOLD PETALS ARE IDEAL FOR SOOTHING ALL MANNER OF SKIN IRRITATIONS.

▼ DRINKING SOOTHING HERBAL TEAS IS A GENTLE WAY TO RELAX BOTH BODY AND MIND.

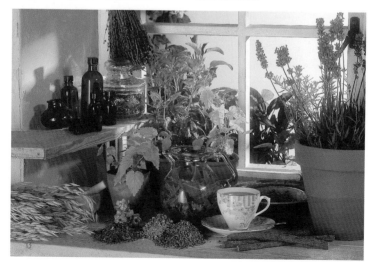

Making teas and tinctures

Flower or herb teas are also called infusions or tisanes. These are made like normal tea, but without adding milk, and are a quick, convenient and refreshing way to extract the goodness and flavour from healing plants.

HEALING TISANES

Many flowers make excellent teas, or tisanes, including chamomile, dandelion, elderflower, hyssop, rose petal, lavender, lime flowers, orange flowers and hibiscus.

Use flowers either singly or in combination, and drink infusions either hot or cold. You need about double the quantity of fresh plant material to dried.

PREPARING TEAS

For best results in retaining the volatile oils, which are the healing essence of the plant, use just-boiled water. Use about 5ml/1 tsp dried or 10ml/2 tsp of fresh flowers or herbs per cup of water.

Place the plant material in a teapot or cafetière (press pot). Pour on water that is off the boil, put the lid on the pot, and steep for up to ten minutes before straining, or pushing down the plunger if using a cafetière. Sweeten with honey, or flavour with lemon or ginger, if desired. Drink three to four doses (500ml/16fl oz) per day. Store infusions in covered containers in the refrigerator for up to 24 hours.

▼ LIMEFLOWERS AND ELDERFLOWERS MAKE A GENTLY SOPORIFIC NIGHT-TIME DRINK.

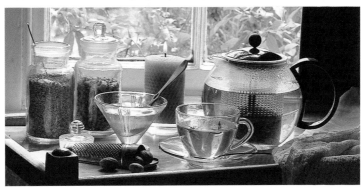

TINCTURES

Sometimes it is more convenient to take a spoonful of medicine rather than make a tea. Tinctures are made by steeping dried or fresh flowers in a mixture of alcohol and water. The alcohol – vodka is a good choice as it contains few additives – dissolves, strengthens and preserves the active ingredients.

HOW TO MAKE A TINCTURE

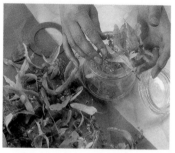

1 Place 115g/4oz dried flowers or herbs or 300g/11oz fresh flowers or herbs in a glass jar.

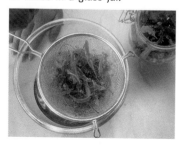

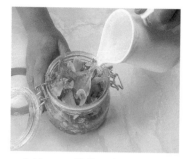

2 Add 250ml/8fl oz/1 cup vodka (30% alcohol or 60% proof).

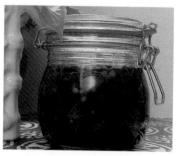

3 Allow the mixture to steep for one month. The best place for this is on a sunny windowsill. Gently shake the jar every day.

4 Strain the mixture and store the prepared tincture in a sterilized, dark glass bottle. When required, you should take a 5ml/1 tsp dosage two to three times a day, diluted in water or fruit juice. Well-made tinctures last for up to two years.

Infused oils and syrups

Active flower ingredients can be extracted in oil and used externally as a massage oil or added to creams and ointments. The two methods of extraction are hot infusion, using simmering heat, and cold infusion, using sunlight.

INFUSED OILS

Hot infusion is preferred for spicy herbs, including ginger or cayenne, and leafy herbs, such as comfrey, chickweed or mullein. The cold method is often used for fresh plants with delicate flowers, such as St John's wort, marigold, chamomile and melilot.

MAKING COLD INFUSED OILS

Pack a glass storage jar with the flowers or leaves of the herb. Pour in a light vegetable oil to cover the herbs, close the jar and shake well. Sunflower and grape

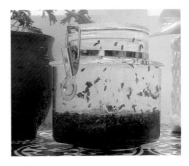

▲ PLACE THE FLOWERS AND THE OIL IN A GLASS JAR AND ALLOW THE CONTENTS TO STEEP FOR ONE MONTH IN A SUNNY LOCATION.

seed oil are good but olive oil is probably the best oil since it will not go rancid.

Allow the jar to stand on a sunny windowsill or in a greenhouse for a month, shaking it every day. The more sunlight there is and the longer the mixture is allowed to steep, the stronger it will be.

Strain the flowers or leaves, using a sieve or muslin bag. For a stronger infusion, renew the flowers in the oil every two weeks and infuse again. Pour the liquid into airtight bottles, label, and store in a cool dark place for up to a year.

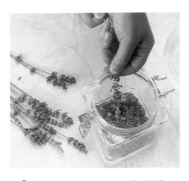

▲ FILL A GLASS STORAGE JAR WITH YOUR CHOSEN FLOWERS OR LEAVES.

Hot-syrup infusions

Since they use honey or unrefined sugar as a sweet preservative, syrups can disguise the taste of bitter plants such as motherwort or vervain. They are thus a good choice of remedy for children. Syrups are soothing in conditions such as sore throats and coughs.

Making syrups

Place 500g/1¼lb sugar or honey into a pan and add 1 litre/ 1¾ pints/4 cups water.

Heat gently and stir until the honey or sugar dissolves fully. Add 130g/4½oz flowers. Heat the ingredients gently for 5 minutes. Turn off the heat and allow the mixture to steep overnight.

Strain and store the syrup in an airtight container in the refrigerator or a cold cupboard. The sugar acts as a preservative so it should keep for up to 18 months.

▼ KEEP PREPARED SYRUPS AND INFUSED OILS IN AIRTIGHT GLASS STORAGE BOTTLES IN A COOL DARK PLACE.

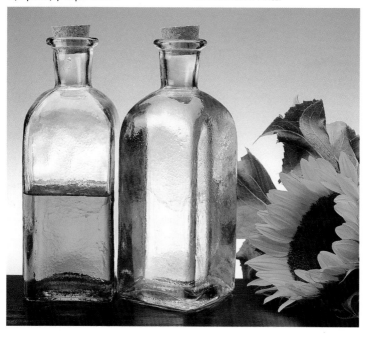

Flower essential oils

Aromatic flowers are so-called because they contain essential oils that carry specific and often therapeutic scents. The use of such oils and aromas to relax, sedate or stimulate has been known for millennia.

FLOWER THERAPY

Aromas have the power to produce emotional reactions within us. A distinctive smell can evoke a long-forgotten memory of a pleasurable or perhaps disturbing experience; it can be an instinctive reaction of attraction or repulsion, or a learned response. We quickly realize that hydrogen sulphide smells bad, like rotten eggs, while a rose is sweet. Some essential oils such as chamomile and lavender are sedating, others such as rosemary and geranium uplifting, but such general qualities can also be modified by our moods.

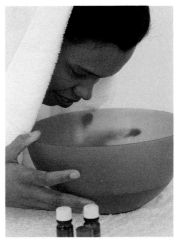

▲ STEAM INHALATION IS A QUICK AND EASY WAY TO ABSORB ESSENTIAL OILS.

WHAT ARE ESSENTIAL OILS?
These are natural, volatile substances, which possess medicinal properties and a distinctive aroma. Essential oils evaporate easily, releasing their scent into the air, as demonstrated when someone brushes against an aromatic plant.

Aromatherapy largely grew out of the perfumery industry, at first with the distillation of essential oils and later with the blending of aromatic oils to yield pleasurable scents. Combining oils is important to aromatherapy, as the effects of individual oils can be magnified in combination. A balanced scent from a blend is likely to be more enjoyable and have a greater therapeutic effect.

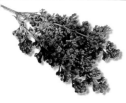

◀ AROMATIC PLANTS CONTAIN ESSENTIAL OILS THAT CAN BE USED TO RELAX, SEDATE, REFRESH OR STIMULATE.

In the early 20th century, the French chemist René-Maurice Gattefosse was working in the family perfumery laboratory, when he badly burned his hand. Plunging it into the nearest liquid, Gattefosse found that the jar of lavender oil he had accidentally used eased the pain, prevented scarring and promoted healing.

Gattefosse then began to examine the therapeutic properties of essential oils, and in 1928 coined the term "aromatherapy" to describe the use of aromatic oils for treating physical and emotional problems.

MASSAGE WITH ESSENTIAL OILS

Essential oils are very concentrated and can damage the skin. Before using them in massage, dilute them with a vegetable carrier oil, such as wheatgerm or almond oil. In general, mix one drop of essential oil with 10ml/ 2 tsp of carrier oil, but use less essential oil if there is any sign of a reaction.

Once diluted, essential oils have a short life, so prepare fresh mixtures in small quantities as needed. Use dry, clean utensils, measuring out about 10ml/2 tsp of vegetable oil into a blending bowl and adding the essential oil one drop at a time. Mix gently.

Body massage is a skill that takes some experience and knowledge of physiology, but essential oils can easily be self-administered for conditions such as chest colds or painful joints. Massage the spot gently with the diluted oils, then rest.

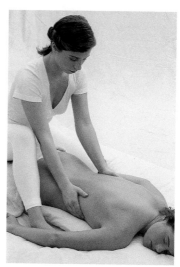

▲ THE NURTURING TOUCH OF MASSAGE IS ENHANCED BY THE AROMA OF ESSENTIAL OILS.

Using essential oils

The powerful ingredients and aromas of essential oils provide therapeutic and pleasant ways to maintain and restore health. Methods of use include inhalations, baths, compresses, massage, potpourris and scented candles.

BUYING AND STORING

Essential oils are sold in dark glass dropper bottles, which protect the contents from light and help in measuring. The oils are highly concentrated, and are diluted for safety and optimum effect. They deteriorate in sunlight, so store in a cool, dark place. Make fresh dilutions as needed, as the oils are volatile. Choose the best-quality oil you can afford, which should guarantee the highest purity.

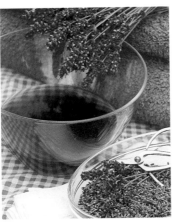

▲ A LAVENDER COMPRESS EASES A HEADACHE.

COMPRESSES

Hot compresses relieve muscle aches and pains: add two drops each of rosemary and marjoram to a bowl of very hot water, dip in a pad of fabric and apply for 30 minutes. Use cold compresses on acute injuries such as sprains, swelling and bruising: add four drops of lavender to a bowl of iced water, dip in a pad and hold in place for 20 minutes.

STEAM INHALATIONS

Using a steam inhalation warms and moistens the mucous membranes, and the use of essential oils helps to open and relax the airways. To relieve colds and sinus problems, pour boiled water into a bowl, add oils and inhale. Try three drops eucalyptus and two drops peppermint for nasal congestion; and four drops lavender, three drops frankincense to relax the airways. Note: take care if you have high blood pressure or asthma.

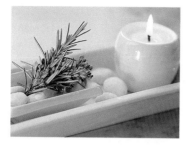

▲ BURN CANDLES SCENTED WITH ESSENTIAL OILS TO CREATE AN EVOCATIVE AMBIENCE.

SCENTING A ROOM

Oil burners consist of a small dish that holds a few drops of essential oil. When gentle heat from a candle is applied under the burner the oil slowly evaporates, producing a long-lasting smell. To fumigate a room, try three to four drops of oils such as eucalyptus, pine or juniper; for alertness, use a couple of drops of rosemary or peppermint; for relaxation, choose ylang ylang or lavender. A bowl of hot water with two drops of lavender oil will moisten the air in an overheated office and add a pleasing scent.

HAND AND FOOTBATHS

A handbath or footbath, consisting of a large bowl with hot water and three to four drops of oil, can relieve migraines and tension

CAUTION

Essential oils are wonderful natural remedies. Their aromatic effects can enhance mood, release tensions and reduce stress. But remember these are highly concentrated substances, to be used with caution. Follow the pointers below, and if in any doubt seek expert advice.

• Never take essential oils internally, unless professionally prescribed.
• Always dilute essential oils – use about 1 part per 100 for massage and only 5 drops in a bath or steam inhalation.
• Follow a "1–2" rule: use one or two oils together, for not more than one or two weeks.
• Seek medical advice before using oils during pregnancy.
• Dilute oils even more for skin problems, and stop use if irritation occurs.
• Take care with asthma or epilepsy, and stop at once if a reaction is experienced.

headaches. Try a lavender and marjoram blend for poor circulation and cold extremities; rosemary and pine for tension and stiffness; and peppermint and lemon to soothe aching hands or feet.

Flower essences

Although people have known of the medicinal benefits of flowers for centuries, modern flower essence therapy began with the work of Edward Bach in 1928. Flower essences are easy-to-use liquid herbal preparations.

A HOLISTIC APPROACH

As people's awareness and healing methods become more holistic, the flower essence philosophy of restoring our health by non-invasive treatment of mental-emotional conditions is gaining ground.

The essences are chosen according to how a person feels about their difficulty, a treatment process that is non-invasive. The compactness of the Bach set makes it a good starting point for people who are beginning their journey into flower essences.

THE SEVEN HELPERS

Gorse	Heather
Oak	Olive
Rock Water	Vine
Wild Oat	

THE 38 BACH REMEDIES

The Seven Helpers are sun-potentized essences for deep, chronic conditions. They are used to support the Twelve Healers.

The Twelve Healers are sun-potentized essences, which correspond to the positive and negative states of 12 basic personality types. These "type essences" support us as we try to find balance and growth, and as we explore inner being throughout our lives.

The second half of the Bach 38 remedy set are essences prepared by the boiling method, and are known as the "New Nineteen Essences". These extend the work of the sun-potentized essences in developing positive spiritual qualities.

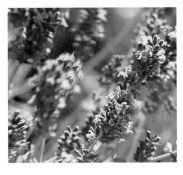

▲ "FLOWERS ARE CONSCIOUS, INTELLIGENT FORCES. THEY HAVE BEEN GIVEN TO US FOR OUR HAPPINESS AND HEALING." LILA DEVI

The Twelve Healers

Negative	Essence	Positive
Restraint	Chicory	Love
Fear	Mimulus	Sympathy
Restlessness	Agrimony	Peace
Indecision	Scleranthus	Steadfastness
Indifference	Clematis	Gentleness
Weakness	Centaury	Strength
Doubt	Gentian	Understanding
Over-enthusiasm	Vervain	Tolerance
Ignorance	Cerato	Wisdom
Impatience	Impatiens	Forgiveness
Terror	Rock Rose	Courage
Grief	Water Violet	Joy

Travelling scents

Flower essences do "travel" quite well beyond their place of production, but some users insist on using essences prepared in their own country. In Australia, the bush essences are well known, while in the USA, Alaskan, Californian and Hawaiian essences are popular. In Europe there are French, Dutch and German essence makers, but the UK still has the largest number of makers and suppliers, including the Bach Centre in Sotwell and Findhorn and Harebell Remedies, Scotland.

The New Nineteen Essences

Aspen	Elm	Mustard	Walnut
Beech	Holly	Pine	White Chestnut
Cherry Plum	Honeysuckle	Red Chestnut	Wild Rose
Chestnut Bud	Hornbeam	Star of Bethlehem	Willow
Crab Apple	Larch	Sweet Chestnut	

Nature's role in preparing essences

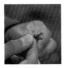

Flower essences are prepared using either of two classical methods; sun potentizing or boiling. In both methods, flowers should be picked from plants growing in a clean, unspoiled environment.

THE DOCTRINE OF SIGNATURES

A belief popularized by Paracelsus nearly 500 years ago, is the doctrine of signatures. It holds that the appearance of a plant relates to its qualities and conveys a message to the healer.

Colour, shape, size and other features all offered insights to the flower healer. The dandelion's yellow colour, for example, suggested a role in healing liver complaints. The patches on lungwort leaves resemble diseased lungs, and the plant was used for bronchitis and tuberculosis.

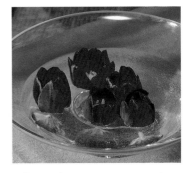

▲ A FLOWER'S ESSENCE ENTERS THE WATER.

This theory was very useful in the development of physical healing, while the Bach tradition has added the vital element of emotional healing.

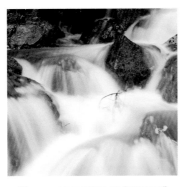

▲ WATER HAS THE POWER TO "MEMORIZE" THE IMPRINT OF FLOWERS.

THE "MEMORY" OF WATER

Edward Bach suggested in the 1930s that the sun is the catalyst which fuses water molecules with the imprint of the flowers used. His claims for potentization were supported by the French scientist Jacques Benveniste, whose experiments showed that water retains the imprint of a substance dissolved in it.

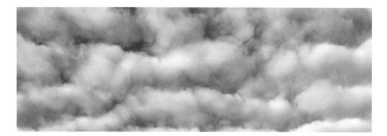

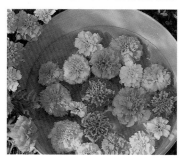

▲ IF CLOUDS APPEAR DURING THE SUN POTENTIZING PROCESS, CONSIDER STARTING AGAIN ON ANOTHER DAY.

SUN POTENTIZING METHOD

Start early in the morning. Fill a thin glass bowl with pure water. Pick your chosen flowers and float them on the water.

Leave the bowl close to where the flowers were growing, in clear sunshine for up to four hours or until the petals fade. The life force of the flowers will pass into the water, which may have changed colour, acquired flavour and feel "zingy" if held. Remove the flowers.

Pour the essence into a clean, clearly labelled bottle. Add an equal amount of brandy. This tincture, now forms the "mother essence", which is diluted later to produce the dosage essence.

▶ FLOAT YOUR FRESHLY PICKED FLOWERS IN A BOWL OF PURE WATER FOR UP TO 4 HOURS.

BOILING METHOD

This is used for flowering trees, such as walnut, which need fire energy to bring out their essence, especially when the blooms are in spring, before the sun is hot.

Instead of picking only blossoms, add twigs too. Place the ingredients in a pan and cover with pure water. Bring to the boil and simmer for 30 minutes. When cool, filter the essence into a bottle with an equal amount of brandy. This tincture is diluted to create flower essence "stock", which can then be diluted for individual use.

Using flower essences internally

Flower essences can be taken internally at any time of day, using a small dropper bottle. A few drops are taken several times a day, depending on the chosen brand, and treatment can be fitted easily into the daily routine.

TAKING ESSENCES

The best times to take the essences are morning and night, when the system is clear, and also before meals. A rhythmical approach like this will give the best results. No advantage is gained by taking a double dose if the previous dose has been forgotten, as taking more than the suggested number of drops is a waste.

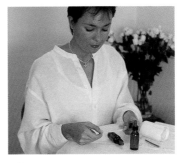

▲ CLEARLY LABEL EACH DOSAGE BOTTLE WITH THE DATE AND CONTENTS LIST.

PREPARING A DOSAGE BOTTLE

1 Almost fill a 30ml/1fl oz dropper bottle with spring water. Add 5ml/1tsp brandy or vodka as a preservative. Use cider vinegar or glycerine if you prefer to avoid alcohol. For babies and animals, omit the preservative, but keep the bottle in the fridge.

2 Add 2 drops of each of your chosen mother essences to the water and brandy mixture. Bang the bottle on your palm to mix.

3 Carry the bottle with you, or prepare several dropper bottles of the essence and have these to hand for different situations.

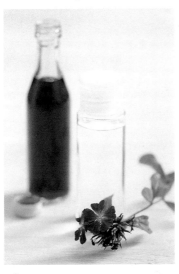

▲ STILL SPRING WATER AND BRANDY FORM THE LIQUID BASE IN DOSAGE BOTTLES.

Dosage is usually 4 drops, four times a day for 3 weeks. Then stop and allow a week to assess the results and decide what to put in a new bottle. Each treatment is based on a four-week cycle.

Alternatively, you may prefer to take essences internally by diluting in a glass of water, adding 2 drops per glass and stirring well. Sip four times a day, and make a fresh batch daily.

The essences can also be taken in pill form. To make the pills, weigh 25g/1oz sugar or lactose pilules in a small jar, add 2 drops of each chosen essence and shake well. Dry the pills on a plate. Chew two a day, with water.

There is no limit on the number of essences that can be taken together. Some herbalists like to use combinations of ten essences, while others will address a core issue using only one essence. Four essences in a treatment bottle is probably a good guideline.

▾ Once the drops are dispersed in a large glass of water, it is virtually impossible to taste the brandy.

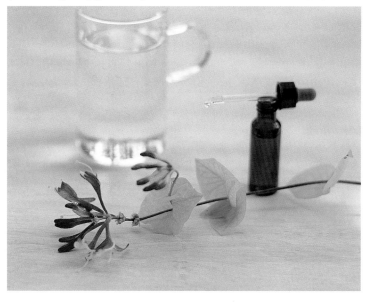

Using flower essences externally

The wide use of flower essences in oils and creams confirms their powerful effect when used externally. Many therapists believe that such usage greatly enhances the effect of the flowers.

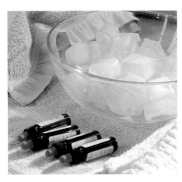

▲ ADD ICE TO A FLOWER COMPRESS TO EASE ACHES CAUSED BY SPRAINS AND SWELLINGS.

SOOTHING COMPRESSES

Lay the compress on any sprain, burn, bite or swelling, and repeat until relief is felt. Seek medical help if appropriate. Fill a bowl with hot or cold water, adding four drops of each chosen essence and four drops of essential oil. Soak a flannel or cotton wool in the water and apply to the affected area.

RELAXING ESSENCE BATHS

Add 12–20 drops of your current dosage essence in a warm bath, or four drops of each chosen mother essence, and swirl the water in a figure of eight pattern to activate the essences. Soak in the bath for 20 minutes and then rest for a further 20 minutes.

HEALING CREAMS

Use a hypoallergenic, non-perfumed cream as a base. Fill a jar with 50g/2oz cream, add four drops of each chosen essence and four drops of an essential oil. Mix with a wooden stick, screw on the jar lid. Apply the finished cream twice daily or as needed.

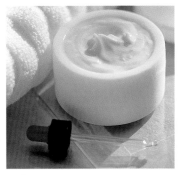

▲ ADD A FEW DROPS OF ESSENTIAL OIL TO YOUR FLOWER ESSENCE CREAM TO ENHANCE ITS HEALING PROPERTIES.

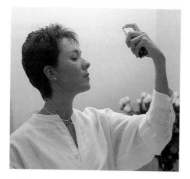

▲ Use flower essence sprays to refresh your mind and uplift your spirits.

Flower essence sprays

Sprays help to cleanse a room of negative energy and refresh stale air. Adding essential oils to flower essences gives an uplifting smell and heightens the healing benefits. Lighter oils such as lavender, geranium and lemon grass work best. Fill a plastic or glass spray bottle with 50ml/2fl oz spring water. Add 10 drops of essential oil and four drops of each chosen flower essence. Shake the bottle and spray as needed.

Flower essence massages

Put four drops of an essential oil and four drops of chosen flower essences into a bottle. Pour in 50ml/2fl oz of cold-pressed almond oil. Shake the bottle to mix and pour the contents into a bowl.

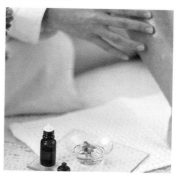

▲ Add flower essence to massage oils.

A FLOWER ESSENCE MASSAGE MIXTURE

- dandelion, for relaxing muscles
- comfrey, also to relax muscles
- chamomile, to relax involuntary muscle spasms
- rock water, to relax the whole body
- valerian, to release stress and tension
- orange hawkweed, to release trauma and energy blocks

Emergency essences

Most people's first introduction to flower essence therapy, and the most well-known of the Bach remedies, is Rescue Remedy. This emergency formula has proved to be helpful for all kinds of stressful situations.

RESCUE REMEDIES

The five classic components in Rescue Remedy are:

- rock rose, for fear
- impatiens, for mental agitation and tension
- cherry plum, for panic and fear of losing control
- clematis, for "faraway" feelings, and unwillingness to face up to a crisis
- star of Bethlehem, for treating panic and shock

Other composite remedies have names such as Five Flower Formula, Emergency Essence, Recovery Remedy, and Calming Essence. All work to restore our emotional and mental balance after shock or trauma, and in "heavy" situations, such as accidents, arguments, bad news, stress at work, or bereavement.

In a crisis, take four drops in a glass of water, sipping slowly. If no water is available,

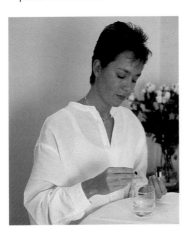

▲ IN A CRISIS ADD FOUR DROPS OF RESCUE REMEDY TO WATER.

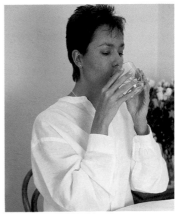

▲ THE QUANTITY OF WATER IS NOT IMPORTANT, BUT SIP SLOWLY.

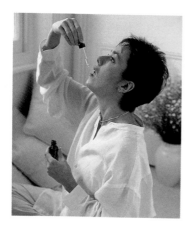

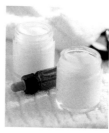

◄ IF NO LIQUID IS AVAILABLE, TAKE DROPS DIRECTLY ON THE TONGUE.

▶ TRY MAKING YOUR OWN RESCUE CREAM.

hypoallergenic base cream and mix. Useful healing additions are up to four drops of lavender or tea tree essential oil.

The cream should be applied at once if bruises, stings, cuts or blisters occur. Apply every two minutes or so for 15 minutes, as the skin absorbs the cream quickly. The liquid remedy should also be taken, or if no cream is to hand, the liquid can even be applied direct to the injury.

take directly on the tongue. Take the remedy every few minutes, as the effect is cumulative.

If a crisis is approaching, make up a dosage bottle: add four drops of Rescue Remedy to a 30ml/1fl oz dropper bottle of spring water. Add 5ml/1 tsp brandy and shake well. Take four times a day or up to 10 times if in need.

Carry a bottle of emergency essence with you at all times, and keep a bottle in the family first aid kit and in the office.

EMERGENCY SPRAYS AND CREAMS

The remedy can also be used as a spray or in cream form. To prepare the cream, add 10 drops of the remedy to 50g/2oz of a

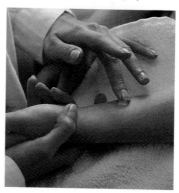

▲ APPLY CREAM IMMEDIATELY IF POSSIBLE.

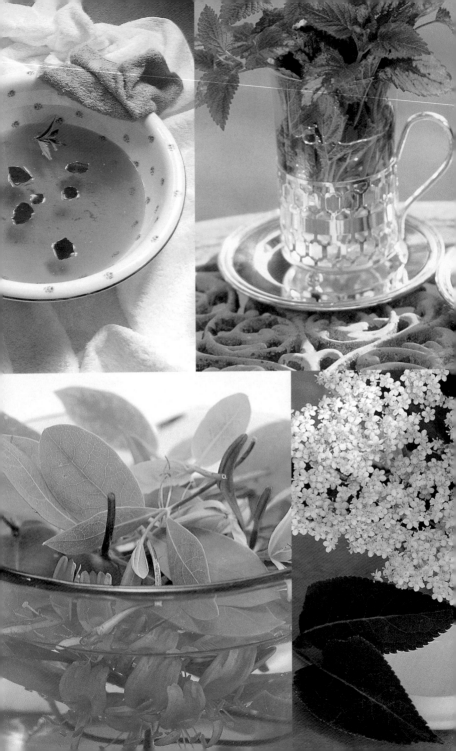

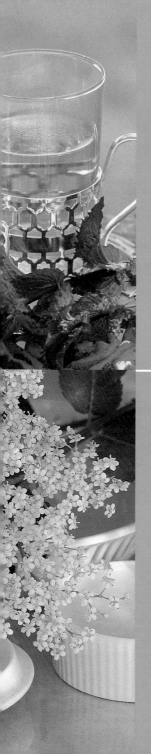

Flower treatments

The flower remedies introduced on the following pages will help you to deal with some of the difficult situations that we all experience from time to time. The recipes are designed to treat some of the most common health problems and conditions. The natural treatments, which include the use of flower essential oils and essences, can be safely self-administered in the home.

Follow the remedies given here, and you should not go wrong. But do not exceed the doses stated, and reduce them if you are pregnant or over 70 years of age. Always be sure to seek professional help if a problem persists or you are uncertain.

Relaxing tense muscles

Sitting in one position too long, as when driving or working at a computer screen, can cause our neck and shoulder muscles to contract. Tiredness, muscle spasm, tension headaches and bad posture may result.

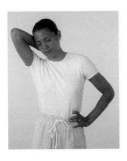

◀ TENSION BUILDING UP IN THE NECK AND SHOULDERS CAUSES STIFFNESS.

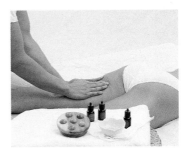

To avoid muscle tension, move frequently, rotating the head or stretching to release the locked muscles. Try to take regular breaks when driving or using computer screens. Massaging stiff muscles with a soothing oil will also help.

▲ MASSAGE WITH A COLD INFUSED FLOWER OIL CAN HELP TO RELEASE AND SOOTHE TENSIONS IN THE MUSCLES.

COLD INFUSED LAVENDER OIL

Home-made infused oils are easy to make and effective in neck or back massages.

Fill a jar with fresh lavender heads and cover with a clear vegetable oil. Steep on a windowsill for two weeks. Shake the jar every day, then strain and bottle. Marjoram and rosemary can be used in the same way.

If using a purchased essential oil of lavender, remember to dilute the oil, with 2 drops of essential oil to 20ml/4 tsp of almond oil, before applying to the skin.

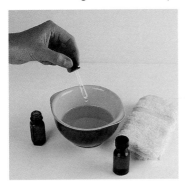

▲ ALWAYS DILUTE ESSENTIAL OILS BEFORE USING ON THE SKIN.

Relieving tension headaches

Headaches and stress go hand in hand with tense muscles. Massaging your head with soothing flower oils, changing the position of the body and taking a scented bath, can all alleviate tension headaches.

LAVENDER OR ROSEMARY BATH

A few drops of essential oil or home-made infused oil in a hot bath will work wonders. To avoid oily smears, try tying a bunch of fresh or dried herbs under the hot tap as you fill the bath.

Lavender or rosemary oil is soothing when rubbed into the head or temples during times of stress. Try mixing 2 drops of essential oil with 5ml/1 tsp of hot or cold water as preferred.

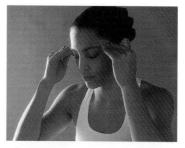

▲ TRY RUBBING LAVENDER OR ROSEMARY ESSENTIAL OIL INTO THE TEMPLES TO EASE A TENSION HEADACHE.

A SOOTHING TEA

Place 2.5ml/½ tsp dried wood betony and 2.5ml/½ tsp dried lavender or rosemary in a cup. Add boiling water, steep for 10 minutes, strain and drink. Drink no more than 2 cups per day.

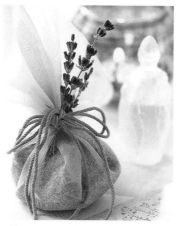

▲ HANG A BAG OF DRIED FLOWERS UNDER A HOT RUNNING TAP FOR A RELAXING AND NATURALLY SCENTED BATH.

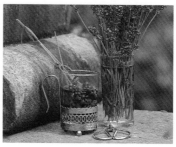

▲ FOR A SOOTHING AND THERAPEUTIC DRINK TRY A LAVENDER TISANE.

Calming anxiety

Anxiety often involves over-excitement and frustration. In such states the body produces adrenaline but in the office or in traffic there is no safe outlet for all this negative energy. Flower remedies can help to calm you down.

ALLEVIATING SYMPTOMS OF ANXIETY

Flower essences and herbal treatments can help tackle symptoms of anxiety such as palpitations, sweating, irritability and sleeplessness.

Use Rescue Remedy in emergencies. If you can take a hot bath, add lavender essential oil

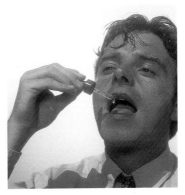

▲ TAKE A FEW DROPS OF RESCUE REMEDY WHEN SUFFERING FROM PANIC ATTACKS.

and relax. St John's wort is an excellent counter to anxiety or depression, especially in winter's dark, cold days.

A TEA FOR ANXIETY

Try combining the nerve tonics and specific remedies listed. Put 5ml/1 tsp of three plants in a tea pot (use only 2.5ml/½ tsp passion flower). Add 600ml/ 1 pint/2½ cups boiling water, leave to steep for 10 minutes. Strain and drink. Take two cups a day for up to 2 weeks.

REMEDIES FOR ANXIETY

• To help calm your nervous system choose: St John's wort; oats; vervain; skullcap; or wood betony. These are all nervine tonics. Choose whichever one suits you best and combine it with a specific remedy for the symptom that troubles you most. Caution: these are powerful herbs, do not exceed the recommended doses (not more than 5ml/1 tsp a day of skullcap and betony, or 2.5ml/½ tsp if in combination).
• To ease palpitations: motherwort or passionflower.
• To reduce sweating: valerian or motherwort.
• To help you sleep: passionflower or valerian.

Fighting nervous exhaustion

We are more susceptible to illness or depression when hard pressed at work or when we face heavy emotional demands. Drinking flower teas is a safe and cheap way to support our nervous systems when stressed.

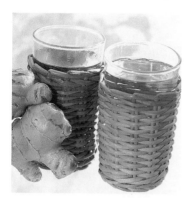

▲ A CUP OF GINGER TEA IS A TASTY TONIC FOR BOOSTING THE NERVOUS SYSTEM.

NERVOUS SYSTEM BOOSTERS
There are a number of flower and herb tonics that can strengthen the nervous system and prevent it running down to the point where nervous exhaustion occurs. Try ginseng, ginger, echinacea or hawthorn.

REVITALIZING TEAS
Mix equal amounts of the following six dried plants that work for nervous exhaustion: oats, licorice, St John's wort, skullcap, borage flowers and wood betony.

Put 15ml/1 tbsp of the mixture into a tea pot, and add 600ml/ 1 pint/2½ cups of boiling water. Steep for 10 minutes and strain. Take one to two cups daily for up to 2 weeks or until the exhaustion passes.

Vervain is another traditional healing plant with a reputation for restoring the nervous system following periods of tension. Vervain's aerial parts, including its stiff, thin stems and small lilac flowers, can be made into a bitter but stimulating tea. It has been used for centuries as an ideal tonic for convalescence from chronic illness.

A well-known restorative tea, for whenever you are tired or stressed, is Earl Grey, which acquires its distinctive flavour from the addition of bergamot oil. Note that the pure essential oil should not be taken internally.

▶ WOOD BETONY RESTORES THE NERVOUS SYSTEM.

Relieving PMS

Many plants have been found to have beneficial effects on the reproductive system, especially in women. Menstrual problems, including cramps, pre-menstrual syndrome and heavy bleeding, can be alleviated by self-treatment.

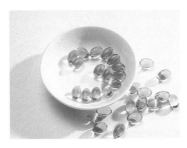

▲ CAPSULES OF EVENING PRIMROSE PROVIDE THE BODY WITH ESSENTIAL FATTY ACIDS, OFTEN LACKING WITH PMS.

Breast tenderness, sore nipples, and fluid retention can often accompany PMS. Lifestyle changes, such as eating extra fresh fruit and vegetables, stopping smoking, taking more exercise, cutting down on salt and processed foods, and relaxing by baths or meditation are all helpful in easing the symptoms.

Good remedies to try are evening primrose capsules or chaste tree (*Agnus castus*) tincture – 12 drops every morning for 3 months, are recommended. Vervain, valerian, lady's mantle and rosemary are also beneficial.

Vervain and rosemary are often taken in infusion form, while valerian is given as tablets or tincture. The name of lady's mantle refers to this plant's traditional value in healing women's conditions, especially in reducing heavy bleeding; it is best avoided during pregnancy.

VERVAIN AND LADY'S MANTLE TEA
Put 5ml/1 tsp each dried vervain and lady's mantle in a pot, and add 300ml/½ pint/1¼ cups boiling water. Steep for 10 minutes, strain and sweeten to taste. Take one cup twice a day from day 14 of the cycle, or 2 weeks after the period begins.

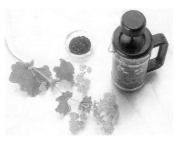

▲ LADY'S MANTLE AND VERVAIN TEA.

Easing periods

Pain during or before periods arises from contraction of the muscles of the womb, which reduces blood flow and causes the muscles to ache. Tisanes and hot compresses can help to ease these menstrual cramps.

Cramp bark (guelder rose) is well-known for reducing spasm, and rosemary is a circulatory stimulant and relaxant.

The leaves of feverfew, lady's mantle, peppermint and valerian have all been used in tisane form to relieve period pain. Among garden flowers, marigold petals in a tisane are known to normalize the menstrual process, and pasque flowers (use only the dried form in tisanes) are a noted relaxant. In each case, infuse 5–10ml/1–2 tsp of the leaves or flowers for up to 10 minutes in boiling water.

A hot-water bottle on the abdomen gives relief, as does a soothing hot herbal compress.

▲ ROSEMARY STIMULATES CIRCULATION.

HOT COMPRESS

Boil 10ml/2 tsp cramp bark in 600ml/1 pint/2½ cups water for 10–15 minutes. Add 10ml/2 tsp dried rosemary. Steep for 15 minutes and strain into a bowl.

Soak a clean cotton cloth or bandage in the liquid. When cool, wring out the cloth. Place the hot compress on the abdomen and relax until it cools.

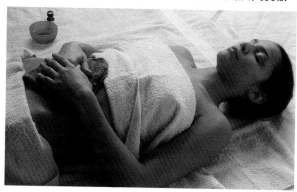

◄ PLACE A HOT COMPRESS ON YOUR ABDOMEN, LIE BACK AND RELAX.

Helping with the menopause

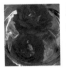

Menopause causes levels of the hormones progesterone and oestrogen to decline. This leads to reduced bone density and adds to the risk of osteoporosis. It is therefore important to support both hormones at this time.

Hormonal changes often lead to unpleasant hot flushes and night sweats. Using plant parts like the berries of chaste tree (*Agnus castus*), lime blossom and sage leaves will help maintain hormone levels, but general vitalizers or tonics are also useful in pepping up a run-down system.

Drinking rose water made by immersing damask rose petals in distilled water is a traditional remedy in the Middle East for alleviating the worst of menopausal symptoms.

TEA FOR HOT FLUSHES
Put 5ml/1 tsp each of motherwort flowers and sage leaves into a cup. Pour on 600ml/1 pint/ 2½ cups of boiling water. Sweeten

with licorice (unless you have high blood pressure). Allow to cool, and sip throughout the day.

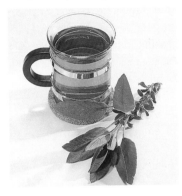

▲ TAKING REGULAR SIPS OF MOTHERWORT AND SAGE TEA THROUGHOUT THE DAY MAY HELP TO EASE MENOPAUSAL HOT FLUSHES.

LIME BLOSSOM TEA
The flowers should be gathered immediately after flowering in midsummer. Collect on a dry day and leave them to dry slowly in the shade. Use as a tincture or make a tisane by mixing a cup of boiling water with 5ml/1 tsp blossom. Leave to steep for up to 10 minutes, then allow to cool. Drink a cup three times a day.

> ### CAUTION
> Sage is a powerful herb and should only be taken for up to 3 weeks at a time. Allow a break of at least a week before taking again.

Lifting depression

Prolonged conditions of stress, anxiety and tension can lead to depression. Physical and mental energy leach away, leaving us vulnerable and unable to recover our equilibrium. There are, however, natural means of helping ourselves.

If external circumstances don't seem to be changing, sometimes all we can do is hang on to our routine until we feel able to cope again. Try to avoid taking pharmaceutical drugs or stimulants at this time. Cooking food may be hard to manage, so this could be the opportunity to buy fresh fruit and vegetables. Keep busy, walk more or do some grounding exercises. Give yourself extra time to relax. Helping others even when we feel depressed is very healing. Flower essences such as mustard, sweet chestnut and gentian, can address our depression, and wild rose and gorse can be used for hopelessness and despair.

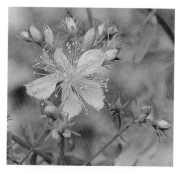

▲ It may be 2 or 3 weeks before St John's wort shows a healing presence.

Restorative tea

Mix equal parts of St John's wort, oatstraw and damiana leaves. Put 10ml/2 tsp in a pot, add 600ml/1 pint/2½ cups boiling water. Steep for 10 minutes and strain. Drink a cup of this tea three times a day.

Caution
You should note that prolonged use of St John's wort may cause skin sensitivity in sunlight.

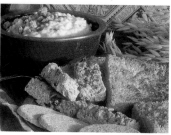

◀ There are many tasty ways in which you can increase your intake of oats as an antidote to depression.

Skin treatments

The skin needs regular cleansing and nourishment to remain healthy. Its condition reflects the general state of your body's health, but many minor skin problems can be improved by the external use of flower remedies.

ABSCESSES

A localized inflamed swelling containing pus is called an abscess. External abscesses on the skin can be treated with hot compresses, but internal abscesses in the mouth or other mucous membranes need qualified medical treatment.

To soothe an external abscess, make a compress by adding no more than 5–6 drops of an essential oil, such as bergamot, chamomile, lavender or tea tree, either separately or combined, to a bowl of boiling water and soak your compress in it. Keep this on the abscess for up to 30 minutes and renew when the compress cools.

ACNE

A common skin condition in adolescence, acne can affect people in later life

◄ WITCH HAZEL

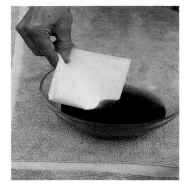

▲ USE A SOFT CLOTH TO MAKE A COMPRESS.

too. It is a sign that the sebaceous glands are producing excess sebum, and the glands and hair follicles are becoming blocked and infected.

Treat with the antiseptic and skin-growth-promoting essential oils tea tree, geranium, lavender or palmarosa, mixing a few drops into a bland carrier oil. Herbal treatments for external use include infusions of elderflower, lavender, marigold or witch hazel. Internally, a decoction of either red clover, burdock or echinacea can tone up the system.

Athlete's foot

This is a fungal infection that causes inflammation and itching between and under the toes, or in the groin. Preventive and controlling measures include scrupulously keeping the feet dry and clean, avoiding synthetic socks and tight-fitting shoes.

Use tea tree or lavender essential oil, or a clove of garlic, rubbed onto the skin twice or more a day. The Indian spice turmeric mixed with a tincture of marigold or myrrh can be applied between the toes.

Skin tonics

Stress and tension cause our muscles to contract, leaving the skin deprived of blood, and often resulting in dryness.

Make up a skin tonic by mixing essential oils into an unperfumed skin cream. Add either 3 drops rose and 3 drops sandalwood, or 4 drops neroli and 2 drops rose to a 25g/1oz pot of skin cream. Arnica, marigold, tea tree and witch hazel can also be applied in paste or cream form.

▸ Rose water is mild and soothing on the skin and also benefits the eyes.

A rose and chamomile facial

Hot water facials open up the pores and leave the skin refreshed and relaxed. Fill a wide bowl with hot water, add 3 drops rose and 4 drops chamomile essential oil. Cover your head with a towel and stay over the bowl for 5 minutes.

Relax for a further 15 minutes. Then apply a toning lotion: for dry skin, mix 75ml/5 tbsp rose water and 30ml/2 tbsp orange flower water; for oily skin, mix 90ml/6 tbsp rose water and 30ml/2 tbsp witch hazel.

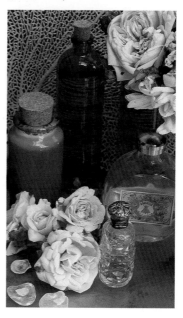

Respiratory ailments

The respiratory tract extends from inside the eyes and nose through the sinuses, throat and airways to the lungs. Flower treatments can combat infection, clear congestion, soothe the membranes and alleviate inflammation.

Avoidance of mucus-forming foods, such as dairy products and refined starches, is advised. So cut out morning cereals and milk, replacing with fruit or fruit juice. Also start taking raw garlic.

CATARRH

When the membranes of nose and throat are irritated, excess mucus may be formed, for example, after a cold. Nasal catarrh occurs higher up in the airways and bronchial catarrh lower down.

A steam inhalation of essential oils, with peppermint, alone or combined with eucalyptus, or tea tree oil helps to loosen mucus and fight infections. For longer-term catarrh, try oil of pine and lavender.

Infusions of peppermint or eucalyptus leaves or chamomile flowers help to ease nasal congestion, as can infusions of the herbs elderflower, golden rod and hyssop.

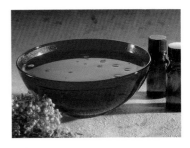

▲ STEAM INHALATIONS HELP TO CLEAR CONGESTION IN THE SINUSES AND CAN AID RECOVERY FROM COLDS AND SORE THROATS.

COLDS

It is difficult to stop a cold virus once it takes hold, and it will usually run its course. Flower treatments, though, can help to relieve symptoms and prevent catarrh or a worse infection taking over. Take plenty of fruit and vitamin C along with other treatments, and cut out mucus-forming foods.

Aromatherapy remedies include baths and steam inhalations. For night-time baths add 10 drops of lavender and 5 drops of cinnamon oil; earlier in the day, use tea tree or eucalyptus (10 drops of each).

A hot infusion of equal parts elderflower, peppermint and yarrow, taken before bedtime will raise the temperature and may sweat out the cold.

Coughs

A cough is a reflex response to irritations or blockages in the airways, so it is better to help the cough rather than suppress it with drugs. Essential oils, such as lavender, thyme and eucalyptus, in a steam inhalation, will do this.

Among many good infusions are marshmallow, thyme, coltsfoot, echinacea and hyssop. For dry coughs, thyme and licorice are recommended, and for mucusy coughs, eucalyptus and licorice.

Sinusitis

The sinus cavities are air spaces in the bones of the skull, around the eyes. Lined with mucous membranes, they are quickly infected by coughs or colds.

Steam inhalations using pine, peppermint, eucalyptus, tea tree, chamomile and lavender essential oils, singly or combined, are all effective at loosening mucus. Catmint, elderflower and golden seal all make strong infusions.

Sore throats

A strong and effective treatment for sore throats and colds is a garlic, ginger and lemon mix: crush a clove of fresh garlic and a similar-sized piece of fresh ginger, adding the juice of a squeezed lemon. Add honey as a sweetener, and mix in hot water. Take up to three times a day.

Steam inhalations of oils such as lavender and thyme can soothe a swollen throat, as can infusions or gargled tinctures of these herbs, or agrimony and sage.

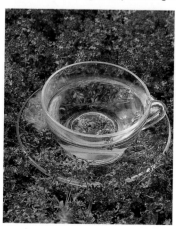

▸ The antiseptic properties of thyme make it an ideal tea for sore throats.

Digestive settlers

 If we are what we eat, we owe it to ourselves to keep our digestive system in good health. The two main roles of plants and flowers in maintaining digestive peace are as stimulants and relaxants.

FOR STOMACH ACHE AND NAUSEA
A cramping stomach pain may be caused by poor digestion or food poisoning, nervous tension or infection. Stomach ache may lead to diarrhoea (see opposite). In general, marigold and garlic are good for fighting digestive infection, while relaxing herbs such as chamomile and cramp bark (guelder rose) will relieve stomach spasms. Nausea can be alleviated by taking frequent sips of a ginger infusion, or 10 drops of tincture diluted in a little water. Lemon will cleanse the stomach.

FOR A NERVOUS STOMACH
You can make a soothing infusion from chamomile, lemon balm and hops, using them either together or separately.

Place 5ml/1 tsp each of chamomile flowers, peppermint and lemon balm into a small tea pot. Fill with boiling water and allow the tea to steep for 10 minutes before straining. Drink the tea three times a day or following meals. Hops can be added to the mixture in the evening to settle the stomach.

▲ MARIGOLD

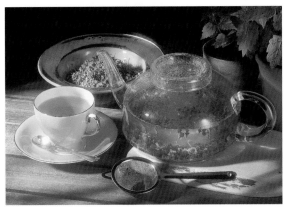

◄ CHAMOMILE TEA IS EFFECTIVE IN MANY DIGESTIVE DISORDERS AND FOR REDUCING NERVOUS TENSION.

A soothing compress

One of the easiest ways to settle an excited stomach is to use an aromatherapy compress, taking the time to relax and allow the soothing essential oils to ease your abdomen.

Measure out 2 drops orange and 3 drops peppermint or 3 drops chamomile and 2 drops orange into a bowl of hot water. Soak a flannel or a bandage in the mixture and place the compress onto the stomach. Lie back and relax for 10 minutes, or longer.

For wind, bloating and colic

Drinking hot teas of catmint, chamomile, ginger or peppermint will help to ease the symptoms. Alternatively, gently massage the abdomen in a clockwise direction with essential oils of chamomile, lemon verbena or peppermint. Dilute the oils at the ratio of 1 drop per 10ml/2 tsp of base oil.

For constipation

One of the most effective methods of self-help is daily clockwise massage of the lower

▶ LEMON BALM MAKES A SOOTHING AND DELICIOUS TEA THAT CALMS THE STOMACH.

CAUTION
Hops are a sedative, so take only at night. Avoid licorice if you have high blood pressure, because it is high in sodium.

abdomen, and this can be performed using 2 drops of oils of lavender, marjoram or rosemary in 5ml/1 tsp of base oil. Alternatively, try chewing on a stick of licorice.

For diarrhoea

An infusion of agrimony or chamomile may help to reduce the impact of tension on the digestive tract. An infusion of meadowsweet may help to settle an acidic stomach. Thyme fights infections and improves digestion generally by settling churning, loose bowels and killing off harmful bacteria.

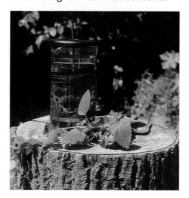

Hangover remedies

Hangovers are not much fun, being a combination of headache, nausea, and depression. Most of these symptoms are associated with the liver, which becomes overloaded and is unable to function properly.

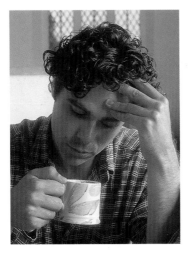

▲ A WARM CUP OF HERBAL TEA WILL PROVIDE COMFORT FOR THE MORNING AFTER.

Headaches and depression are dealt with elsewhere. In both cases traditional plant treatments remain good alternatives to drugs.

Fresh ginger made into a tea, with honey and lemon to taste, is a good antidote to nausea. Dandelion coffee, made from the plant's roots, or the leaves and flowers sometimes used for salads, will help restore the liver. Both ginger and dandelion have strong tastes, but a vigorous defence is needed to deal with the alcohol assault and restore our system to balance and good health.

Bitter plants, such as lavender, vervain and dandelion, are good for stimulating the liver, helping detoxify it and lift the spirits generally. Rather than "the hair of the dog" (another drink), try a morning-after tea, with plenty of vitamin C and water to rehydrate the system. When you do drink alcohol, drink water alongside it to literally dilute the poisoning effect on your system.

A MORNING-AFTER TEA
Put 5ml/1 tsp dried vervain and 2.5ml/½ tsp lavender flowers into a pot, and add 600ml/1 pint/2½ cups boiling water. Allow to steep for 10 minutes, strain and sweeten with honey. Sip this tea often until you begin to feel better. ▲ LAVENDER

Tonics for convalescence

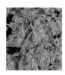

After an illness when the symptoms have gone, try to allow proper time for the body to recover. Disease depletes our immune system and makes us more vulnerable to post-viral syndrome or a recurrence of the original problem.

The old-fashioned concept of a tonic has its place here. For example, oatstraw and St John's wort flowers support the nervous system, vervain stems and flowers promote relaxation, and licorice root and borage flowers restore the effectiveness of the adrenal glands.

An infusion of thyme leaves will help restore vitality and reduce the chances of colds and flu, while ginseng is a tried-and-tested tonic for old age as well as convalescence. Ginseng is considered a strong tonic, and it is advised to avoid caffeine while using it. All these tonics should be taken for a few weeks or even a couple of months after the illness.

Vitamin C supplements or large amounts of citrus fruit taken for several weeks after your illness help in convalescence. Rest is important, as is a nourishing diet. Alfalfa or mung bean sprouts are a handy and cheap source of fresh vitamins and minerals.

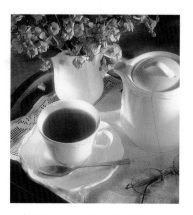

▲ A TONIC WILL AID YOUR RECOVERY.

A TONIC TEA

Put 2.5ml/½ tsp each of oatstraw, vervain stems and flowers, St John's wort flowers, borage leaves and licorice root into a tea pot. Add boiling water, flavouring with peppermint to taste. Let steep for 10 minutes, strain. Drink three or four cups, warm, each day for at least 3 weeks. Avoid licorice if you have high blood pressure.

Enhancing sleep and relaxation

Flowers and herbs are unsurpassed in their ability to help us sleep and to relax. Sedative herbs aid in relaxation when taken at night, and stimulating herbs are used when we are overstimulated and there is nervous exhaustion.

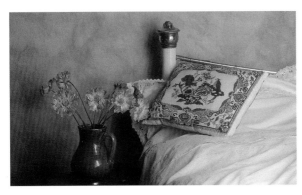

◄ A SOFT FLOWER PILLOW, WHETHER MADE OR BOUGHT, IS A GOOD FIRST STEP IN IMPROVING YOUR SLEEP ENVIRONMENT.

Sedative flowers often used in infusions are, in ascending order of strength, chamomile, lime, lavender and passion flower. Infusions in the evenings are relaxing, as are baths (see opposite). A hop or herbal pillow works for some people. The important thing is to take some time to relax and unwind, doing something peaceful after a day's work, such as gentle exercise, meditation, reading, yoga or tai chi.

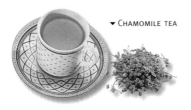

▼ CHAMOMILE TEA

SLEEPY-TIME TEA

Put 5ml/1 tsp each of dried chamomile, lemon balm and vervain in a pot, and pour on 600ml/ 1 pint/2½ cups boiling water. Steep for 10 minutes. Strain and drink a cup after supper and another before going to bed.

For a stronger blend, add a decoction of 5ml/1 tsp valerian root or 2.5ml/½ tsp dried hops or Californian poppy. Never take more than 2.5ml/½ tsp hops per day.

Bath therapy

A hot bath, with the aroma of exotic flowers, and perhaps a candle and soothing music is an inexpensive, easily arranged yet unsurpassed relaxation therapy we can enjoy in our own homes.

In addition to quick baths or showers to get clean, we should often award ourselves the time for a relaxing bath, using essential oils to make our bathtimes particularly healing experiences. Pour 5 drops of an oil into the bath water just before you are ready to enter. This will form a thin film on the surface of the water, and the oil will be easily absorbed by the skin, whose pores are being opened up by the heat. Breathing in the aroma is also therapeutic for both the mind and body.

A refreshing morning bath is produced by adding 3 drops bergamot and 2 drops geranium oil. For an unwinding evening bath, blend 3 drops lavender and 2 drops ylang ylang. For aching muscles at any time, use 3 drops marjoram and 2 drops chamomile essential oils.

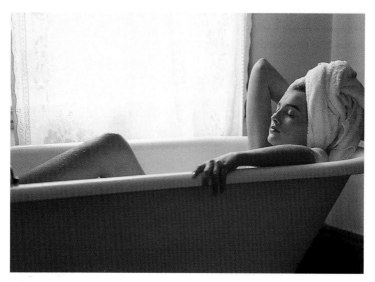

▲ TREAT YOURSELF TO A LONG BATH WITH ESSENTIAL OILS.

Healing flowers directory

This directory features 60 of the best-known healing flowers, with brief descriptions and distributions, followed by their uses and possible restrictions. Take care when using flowers internally, and consult a qualified herbalist if in any doubt.

Achillea millefolium, YARROW
A pungent perennial herb with flat, whitish or pink flowerheads 15 – 30cm (6 – 12in) above feathery leaves. The essential oil can treat catarrh, the bitter-tasting infusion sweats out colds and fevers; used externally for wounds, nosebleeds and as a skin toner (Achillea refers to the soldiers of the legendary Achilles using yarrow to staunch their wounds in battle).

Agrimonia eupatoria, AGRIMONY
Perennial herb with yellow flower spikes, 30–60cm (1–2ft) high. Dried flowers make an anti-inflammatory, anti-bacterial, astringent infusion; used internally for sore throats, catarrh, diarrhoea, cystitis, urinary infections; external lotion for wounds, staunching bleeding. Also a Bach flower essence.

Althaea officinalis, MARSHMALLOW
Hardy perennial, to 1–1.2m (3–4ft) high, with pale pink flowers. Flowers and roots are famed for soothing, sweet mucilage, and as lozenges relieve inflamed gums and mouth, gastric ulcers and bronchial infections. Externally, the flowers soothe inflamed skin. The modern candy confection no longer contains the herb.

Anemone pulsatilla, PASQUE FLOWER
A hardy perennial, 15cm (6in) in height, with exquisite purple-blue flowers and yellow anthers. Used for treating cramps, PMS and menstruation, also male reproductive problems; usually taken in homeopathic rather than fresh form, as the plant is toxic. A word of caution: you should avoid taking pasque flower remedies during pregnancy.

Arnica montana, Arnica

An alpine perennial, 30–60cm (1–2ft) tall, with yellow, daisy-like flowers. Both therapeutic and toxic. For use internally, take only in homeopathic doses, for shock and pain; externally, use as a cream, for bruises and sprains.

Artemisia absinthium, WORMWOOD

Perennial shrub, 3ft (1m) high, with hairy stems and aromatic, downy grey-green leaves. One of the bitterest plants known (*absinthium* means "without sweetness"), it is a strong tonic for the digestive system but toxic in excess. Useful for anaemia, easing wind and in recuperation.

Borago officinalis, BORAGE

Hairy annual, 60cm (2ft) high, with large leaves and mauve-blue star-shaped flowers. Aerial parts used externally on inflamed skin, but contain toxins and use is restricted in some countries. Essential oil is safe, and good for hormonal problems and PMS.

Calamintha nepeta, CALAMINT

A bushy perennial mint, 30–60cm (1–2ft) high, with tubular, pink-mauve flowers. Leaves and flower tops are used as a stimulating tea or as a tonic or infusion for settling wind and indigestion. Avoid use during pregnancy.

Calendula officinalis, CALENDULA

The marigold, or pot marigold, a cheerful, low-growing annual to 50cm (20in) high, with distinctive orange-yellow petals. Wonderful herb, antiseptic, anti-inflammatory, anti-bacterial and anti-fungal. A soothing ointment for irritated skin, eczema, sunburn, bites; good addition to hand and face cream.

Carthamus tinctorius, SAFFLOWER

Hardy annual, 1m (3ft) in height, with shaggy, thistle-like red-yellow flowerheads. A tea, infused from the flowers, induces perspiration and reduces fevers. Infusions are used externally for bruises, skin irritations and measles. Avoid use during pregnancy.

Centaurea cyanus,
CORNFLOWER
Annual, 20 – 80cm (8 – 32in) tall, with bright blue shaggy flowerheads. Flowers used traditionally to make eyewashes for tired or strained eyes. Petals make a bitter tonic, the seeds a mild laxative for children.

Chamaemelum nobile,
CHAMOMILE
Evergreen perennial 30cm (1ft) high, with feathery leaves. White daisy-like flowers have yellow centres. Antiseptic, anti-inflammatory, soothing and sedative as infusion or essential oil. Used for nausea, indigestion, aiding sleep and menstruation, and as ointment for stings and bites.

Citrus aurantium,
BITTER ORANGE
Evergreen tree, up to 8m (26ft) in height, shiny leaves and fragrant white flowers, bitter "Seville" orange fruits. Essential oil of neroli made from the flowers, oil of petitgrain from leaves and twigs, oil of orange from rind. Do not take oils internally. Rich in vitamins A, B and C, tonic and calming effects.

Cnicus benedictus,
HOLY THISTLE
Annual, 65cm (26in) high, with red, hairy stems, spiny leaves and yellow flowers. Leaves and tops used, with bitter, antiseptic, antibiotic qualities. Infusion or tincture taken as a tonic, for fevers and settling stomach.

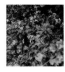

Crataegus laevigata,
HAWTHORN
Common deciduous shrub/small tree, grows up to 8m (26ft) tall. It has thorny branches, white, scented flowers in spring (May blossom) and red, globe-shaped fruit, known as haws, in autumn. Bioflavonoid content makes it a valuable, slow-working "food for the heart". It regulates its rhythm and lowers blood pressure – especially good for treating hypertension. It is said to be gradual in effect and well tolerated by the body.

Crocus sativus,
SAFFRON CROCUS
A perennial crocus, with round corm. In autumn it produces lilac flowers with purple veins, yellow anthers and three red styles. The styles are dried to make saffron, which is known to have digestive properties, improve circulation and reduce high blood pressure. It is used widely in cooking and is a rich source of vitamin B2.

Echium vulgare,
VIPER'S BUGLOSS
A bushy and bristly biennial, 60–90cm (2–3ft) tall, with speckled stems, prickly leaves and spires of violet-blue flowers. The doctrine of signatures held that, because it resembled a snake's skin and tongue, it must be an antidote to adder bite or other poisons. It is toxic if taken internally, but has skin-healing properties.

Eschscholzia californica,
CALIFORNIA POPPY
Annual or perennial poppy, 60cm (2ft) high, with bright orange, yellow or pink flowers, native to western North America. It is a sedative plant that relieves pain and is taken internally as an infusion, for anxiety, nervous tension and insomnia. Good for children, for bedwetting or sleeping problems.

Eupatorium cannabinum,
HEMP AGRIMONY
A hard and woody perennial, 1.2m (4ft) tall, with red stem and pink-white flowers (a local name was "raspberries and cream"). Whole plant used, as a diuretic and for kidneys, as a tonic and for flu-like illnesses. Alkaloid content means caution necessary in internal use. Applied externally to ulcers and sores.

Euphrasia officinalis,
EYEBRIGHT
An annual, semi-parasitic herb. It is 5–30cm (2–12in) tall and grows on grasses. White flowers lipped with yellow throats and purple veins. Infusion used externally as bath for sore or itchy eyes, skin irritations; internally for bad colds.

Filipendula ulmaria,
MEADOWSWEET
Tough, herbaceous perennial, 1–1.2m (3–4ft) tall, with dense, fluffy, creamy flowers. Leaves and flowers used as infusion for heartburn, excess acid and gastric ulcers, and rheumatism, arthritis and urinary infections. Was formerly used to make aspirin. Safe remedy for children with diarrhoea and upset stomachs.

Galega officinalis,
GOAT'S RUE
A bushy and hardy perennial, up to 1.5m (5ft) tall, with pea-type mauve, white or bicoloured flower spikes. Has sedative properties and infusions are taken for irritability and insomnia. A diuretic, it can improve liver function and has a tonic effect on the system.

Galium odoratum or *Asperula odorata,*
SWEET WOODRUFF
Spreading perennial, 40cm (16in) tall, with spear-shaped leaves and small, white star-shaped flowers. Used as infusion for soothing nerves and insomnia, as a diuretic, to improve liver function and for varicose veins. Caution: avoid use during pregnancy.

Geranium maculatum
CRANESBILL
Hardy perennial, up to 75cm (30in) tall, with round, purplish-pink flowers, native to North America. Whole plant dried for infusions, powders and tinctures; used as astringent to control bleeding and discharges, for diarrhoea and haemorrhoids; externally for wounds and as gargle for sore throats and mouth ulcers.

Geum urbanum,
WOOD AVENS
A hardy perennial, 20–60cm (8–24in) high, with small, five-petalled yellow flowers. Flowers used in infusions, roots in decoctions, for digestive upsets and as a tonic, for sore gums and mouth inflammations; externally for haemorrhoids. The old name, herb bennet, recalls "benedict" (blessed) and the belief that it repelled evil spirits.

Helianthus annuus
SUNFLOWER
Tall annual, up to 3m (10ft) high, with large flowerheads up to 30cm (1ft) across, yellow ray and brown disc florets. Whole plant used for extracts and tincture, seeds for commercial vegetable oil. Good source of vitamin E (an antioxidant) and polyunsaturates (maintain cell membranes and lower blood cholesterol).

Hypericum perforatum,
ST JOHN'S WORT
Hardy perennial, 30–60cm (1–2ft) tall, with small leaves, five-petalled yellow flowers, used as cream, tincture, infused oil. Calms anxiety states, reduces nervous tension; an antiseptic, promotes healing on skin, muscles; antidepressant. Can cause sensitivity in sunlight; use controlled by law in Australia.

Hyssopus officinalis,
HYSSOP
Semi-evergreen and bushy perennial, some 60–90cm (2–3ft) high, flowers in dense blue-pink spikes. Leaves, flowers used traditionally as a cure-all infusion, as an expectorant, for promoting sweating and as an anti-catarrhal and anti-bacterial. Its essential oil is restricted in some countries.

Jasminum officinale,
JASMINE
Evergreen rambler, to 6m (20ft), with sweet-scented white flowers. Flowers are used as a calming infusion; the essential oil is anti-depressant, euphoric and relaxing, used externally on dry skin and in the bath or massage oil; not to be taken internally.

Lavandula angustifolia,
LAVENDER
Cultivated for so long that it now has numerous hybrids. Common lavender is 60–90cm (2–3ft) tall, with small purple flowers, used in perfumes, cooking, inhalations and decoration. The first aromatherapy oil, it remains an excellent first aid remedy for skin problems, headaches and nervous digestion.

Leonurus cardiaca,
MOTHERWORT
A hardy, pungent perennial, up to 1.2m (4ft) tall, with mauve-pink, double-lipped flowers. Flowering tops used in infusions and tinctures, with calming effect on the heart and for palpitations; suitable for period pain and PMS, but despite original usage it is no longer given to pregnant women.

Lilium candidum,
MADONNA LILY
Perennial, up to 1–1.5m (3–5ft) high, with racemes of 5–20 fragrant, white trumpet-shaped flowers with yellow anthers. Juice from roots and flowers used externally in ointments for burns, and skin inflammations; flowers made into perfumed essence.

Lonicera periclymenum,
HONEYSUCKLE
Hardy climber, up to 7m (23ft), with fragrant, creamy-white/yellow two-lipped flowers, followed by poisonous red berries. Little used now in Western herbal medicine, the leaves were favoured as an expectorant, the bark as a diuretic and flowers for asthma. A Bach remedy for nostalgia.

Lycopus europaeus,
GIPSYWEED
A perennial mint-like herb, but without the aroma. Grows to 60cm (2ft) tall, with toothed leaves and small mauve flowers. An astringent and sedative, once used to treat haemorrhaging, palpitations and menstrual problems. Its black dye, used by gypsies to darken their skin, gave the common name.

Lythrum salicaria,
PURPLE LOOSESTRIFE
A perennial, up to 0.6cm–1.5m (2–5ft) high, with erect stems and crimson-purple flowers. Astringent, used in infusions, decoctions and ointments, internally for diarrhoea (including nursing babies) and heavy menstruation, externally for soothing wounds, eczema. Classified as noxious in some countries and imports forbidden.

Marrubium vulgare, HOREHOUND

Hardy perennial, 60cm (2ft) tall, nettle-like leaves, small white flowers, a common weed (controlled by law in Australia and New Zealand). From Egyptian and Biblical times, stems used as a bitter infusion for non-productive coughs, colds and chest infections. Also a gargle and cough candy.

Melilotus officinalis, MELILOT

An erect, straggly biennial, 0.6cm–1.2m (2–4ft) high, with ridged stems and yellow, honey-scented flowers in spikes (the name means honey-lotus). Dried flowering stems used in infusion or tincture as sedative and anti-inflammatory. Used to treat insomnia, headaches, flatulence and menopause. Caution: improperly dried plant is toxic.

Melissa officinalis, LEMON BALM

A bushy perennial, 30–80cm (12–32in) high, with pungent, rough, toothed leaves and small pale yellow flowers. Infusions are sedative and soothing. They are good for treating headaches, indigestion, nervous tension and depression. Externally, poultice or creams soothe skin problems.

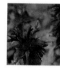

Monarda didyma, BERGAMOT

An aromatic hardy perennial, 40–90cm (16–36in) high, with red or mauve flowers. Native of North America, made into Oswego tea by early European settlers. Leaves and flowers in infusion aid digestion. Bergamot essential oil, extracted from the bergamot orange, *Citrus bergamia*, is used to flavour Earl Grey tea.

Nepeta cataria, CATMINT

A hardy perennial mint, 30–90cm (1–3ft) tall, with coarse leaves and whitish-mauve flowers. Catmint is irresistible to cats. An anti-inflammatory and a mild sedative. Leaves, flowers and stems make an infusion for feverish colds; used externally for cuts and bruises. Mild enough for children.

Oenothera biennis,
EVENING PRIMROSE
Not related to the primrose, but is named because flowers open in the evening. Erect biennial, to 1.5m (5ft) tall, with bright yellow blooms; native of North America. Seeds pressed for oil used for boosting immune system and hormones. Taken internally for PMS, menopause, allergies; externally for skin tone.

Origanum majorana,
SWEET MARJORAM
Half-hardy aromatic perennial, to 60cm (2ft) tall, with small lilac-pink flower clusters. A warming, relaxing, antiseptic herb, taken as an infusion to treat nervous tension, headaches, insomnia, colds, digestive complaints and painful periods. The essential oil is applied to stiff muscles, and joints.

Passiflora incarnata,
PASSION FLOWER
A hardy, tropical perennial climber, to 8m (26ft), creamy-white to lavender intricate flowers. Leaves and flowers dried for infusions, tinctures and tablets; a gentle sedative and tranquillizer for nervous conditions and insomnia.

Pelargonium graveolens,
GERANIUM
A bushy aromatic perennial, also called rose geranium, to 1m (3ft) high, with pink flowers. Native to southern Africa, now a universal house plant. Contains a volatile oil used in perfumery industry, and dried leaves go into various scents and aromatics. Astringent, antidepressant, good in teas for nervous tension and exhaustion.

Primula veris,
COWSLIP
A spring perennial with stems rising 15–20cm (6–8in), bearing cluster of tubular yellow flowers. Becoming rare in the wild, but flowers and roots used traditionally as sedative infusion for children and as expectorant; taken for insomnia, chronic respiratory tract infections and rheumatism. Avoid in pregnancy or if allergic to aspirin.

Primula vulgaris, PRIMROSE
A perennial, up to 15cm (6in), with clusters of saucer-shaped, pale yellow flowers in early spring. Similar properties to cowslip. Flowers (cultivated only, as wild form is rare and protected) used as infusion for calming anxiety, in insomnia and respiratory tract problems.

 Prunella vulgaris, SELFHEAL
Aromatic perennial herb, to 50cm (20in) tall, with violet, two-lipped florets. Aerial parts dried for infusions, tinctures and ointments. Antibacterial and astringent, used formerly as a wound herb, to stop bleeding, for bites, bruises, sore throats and inflamed gums.

 Rosa gallica var. *officinalis*, ROSE
Deciduous bush, to about 1.5m (5ft), multiple varieties. Used medicinally since antiquity (called Apothecary's rose), as water, ointment, syrup, vinegar, conserve, candies etc., mainly now for flowers, essential oil ("attar of roses"). A Bach remedy. Mildly sedative, antidepressant, aphrodisiac; rose water for sore eyes; hips for vitamin C.

 Rosmarinus officinalis, ROSEMARY
An evergreen shrub, to 2m (6ft), with woody branches, aromatic, needle-like leaves and small pale blue flowers. Leaves and flowers make infusion for colds, flu, headaches; a tincture for depression, nervous tension; essential oil for massages to relieve rheumatic, muscular pain and in baths for tiredness. Avoid in excess during pregnancy.

 Sambucus nigra, ELDER
Small deciduous tree, to 10m (33ft) tall, with creamy umbels of musky white flowers and clusters of black fruits later. Often grows as weed. Infusions of flowers taken for colds, sinusitis, hayfever; berries make cough syrups. Leaves boiled for an insecticide, flowers used for home-made skin toners. Note: leaves are toxic.

Solidago virgaurea,
GOLDEN ROD
Hardy perennial, up to 1m (3ft) tall, with branched stems and profuse spikes of yellow flowers. Antioxidant, diuretic and astringent. Leaves and flowers make lotions, ointments and poultices used externally for wounds, bites and rashes; internally, infusions used for urinary problems and Candida.

Stachys officinalis,
BETONY
Hardy perennial, up to 60cm (2ft) high, with magenta-pink flowers. Leaves and flowers used historically in infusion, ointment and lotion form for headaches. Still applicable today, also for anxiety, PMS and "nerves", but not during pregnancy. Externally, good for cuts and bruises. Toxic in excess.

Tilia cordata, LIME
A hardy, deciduous tree, up to 25m (82ft) high, with heart-shaped leaves and fluffy pale yellow flowers. New-opened flowers dried for linden teas, which are soothing and sweat-inducing. Mix with honey and lemon for colds, catarrh, fevers, anxiety and nervous palpitations. Reduces high blood pressure.

Trifolium pratense,
RED CLOVER
Short-lived perennial, grows up to 20–60cm (8–24in) in height, with circular pink flowerheads. Used herbally, with infusion of blossoms for coughs and eczema and externally applied on breast cancers, in skin conditions for ulcers, burns and sores. Formerly used for cataracts as white leaf halo suggested this "signature".

Tropaeolum majus,
NASTURTIUM
Half-hardy annual, stems, 3m (10ft) high, with circular leaves and yellow-orange single flowers. Native to Peru, used in Andean herbal medicine as disinfectant and expectorant. Infusions taken for urinary infections and clearing nasal, bronchial catarrh; fresh leaves and flowers are high in vitamin C content.

Tussilago farfara,
COLTSFOOT
A small creeping perennial, to 15–20cm (6–8in) high, flowers bright yellow, emerging in early spring. Leaves or flowers are tonics, soothing to mucous membranes and an ancient remedy for sore chests, used in infusion for coughs; externally, as compress or paste for sores, ulcers, bites. Not suitable for use during pregnancy or for children.

Verbena officinalis, VERVAIN
Hardy, rather straggly perennial with erect, branched stem and lobed dull green, slightly hairy leaves. Small, pale-lilac flowers sparsely arranged in terminal spikes. Vervain has mildly sedative and hypnotic properties and is taken in infusions for nervous exhaustion, anxiety, insomnia, tension headaches and migraine. Also for disorders associated with the stomach, kidneys, liver and gall bladder. Externally it is used in compress and lotions for skin complaints and as a gargle for sore gums and mouth ulcers.

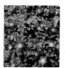

Vinca major,
GREATER PERIWINKLE
Trailing evergreen perennial, to 45cm (18in), glossy dark-green leaves and violet blue flowers. Leaves and flowering stems, processed to extract an alkaloid, dilates blood vessels and reduces blood pressure. Caution: all parts are poisonous, self-treatment not advised.

Viola odorata, SWEET VIOLET
Low-growing hardy perennial, up to 15cm (6in) tall, basal rosette of leaves and single, drooping purple or white spring flowers. Flowers yield an aromatherapy essential oil, other parts a gentle infusion or syrup for coughs, colds and rheumatism.

Viola tricolor,
WILD PANSY
Annual or perennial, growing to 38cm (15in), with violet, yellow and white triangular flowers. Also called heartsease, in reference to its older use as a heart tonic. Used in infusion as expectorant for coughs and colds; used externally to treat skin complaints.

index

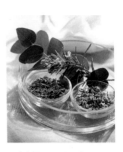

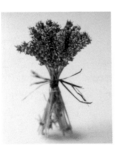